YOUR KNOWLEDGE HAS VALUE

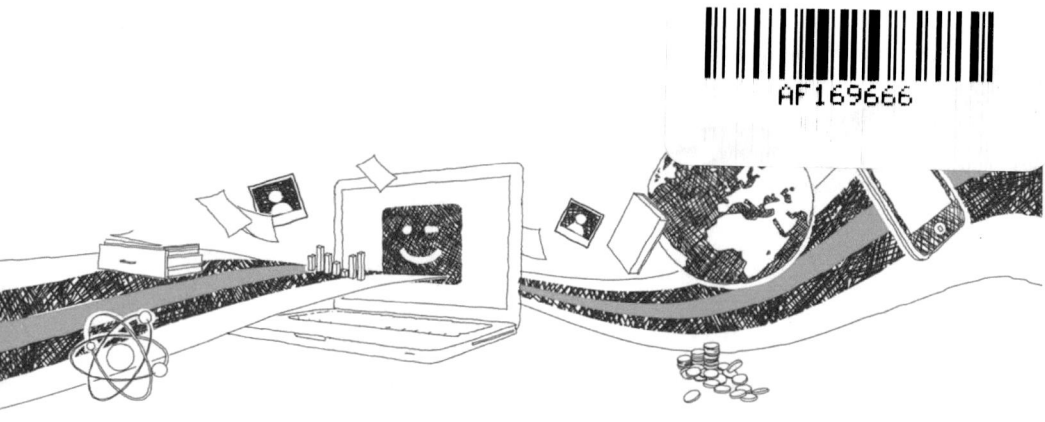

- We will publish your bachelor's and master's thesis, essays and papers

- Your own eBook and book - sold worldwide in all relevant shops

- Earn money with each sale

Upload your text at www.GRIN.com
and publish for free

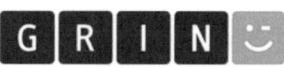

Bibliographic information published by the German National Library:

The German National Library lists this publication in the National Bibliography; detailed bibliographic data are available on the Internet at http://dnb.dnb.de .

This book is copyright material and must not be copied, reproduced, transferred, distributed, leased, licensed or publicly performed or used in any way except as specifically permitted in writing by the publishers, as allowed under the terms and conditions under which it was purchased or as strictly permitted by applicable copyright law. Any unauthorized distribution or use of this text may be a direct infringement of the author s and publisher s rights and those responsible may be liable in law accordingly.

Imprint:

Copyright © 2016 GRIN Verlag, Open Publishing GmbH
Print and binding: Books on Demand GmbH, Norderstedt Germany
ISBN: 9783668489745

This book at GRIN:

http://www.grin.com/en/e-book/368335/contemporary-nursing-issues-legal-and-ethical-issues-in-healthcare

Leonard Kahungu

Contemporary Nursing Issues. Legal and Ethical Issues in Healthcare

GRIN Publishing

GRIN - Your knowledge has value

Since its foundation in 1998, GRIN has specialized in publishing academic texts by students, college teachers and other academics as e-book and printed book. The website www.grin.com is an ideal platform for presenting term papers, final papers, scientific essays, dissertations and specialist books.

Visit us on the internet:

http://www.grin.com/

http://www.facebook.com/grincom

http://www.twitter.com/grin_com

Running Head: LEGAL AND ETHICAL ISSUES IN HEALTHCARE

Legal and Ethical Issues in Healthcare

Leonard Kahungu

Contemporary Nursing Issues

LEGAL AND ETHICAL ISSUES IN HEALTHCARE

Legal and Ethical Issues in Healthcare

End-of-life Issues

In patient-centered care, end of life is one of the most important aspects of health care systems. Advanced nursing and medical studies have increased the knowledge regarding the process of dying, giving the humans the privilege of selecting the method, location and approximate period of death. Similarly, intervening in the death process can also increase the lifespan of a person, even when there is little hope of living longer or full recovery. Despite the vast knowledge of mortality, there are still contemporary end-of-life issues that remain contradictory among different cultures.

One of the primary reasons why end-of-life issues have not been sufficiently addressed is because of different values held by various religions, cultures and beliefs. Life is highly valued in most of the cultures and religious groups. It is believed that only the Supreme Being is allowed to take, give or control how long a person is supposed to live. Moreover, there are high emotions that are often attached to people since the death of a person means complete extraction of the physical presence of a person. Thus, such emotions and cultural beliefs are the major hindrances that cripple the smooth readdress of end-of-life (Guido, 2014).

Passive Euthanasia and Physician-Assisted Suicide

Physician-assisted suicide is used to describe a process where a registered general practitioner provides the means of dying to the patient. This is often achieved through the prescription of certain substances. The patient administers the rather medication to him or herself, initiating the death procedure (Dworkin, 2008). In some cases, the physician may act directly in the administration of the extreme medication to terminate the life of a person. On the other hand, allowing patients to die, or passive euthanasia involves withholding medication, treatment or withdrawing life support machines with the primary aim of achieving death of a person. There are, however, strict procedures that must be observed so as to reduce any liabilities to the individuals or practitioners involved in the process.

Allowing a person to die naturally does not interfere with the death process. In fact, it can be termed as a natural death, when medication or further treatment is withheld to allow nature take its course. On the other hand, physician-assisted suicide quickens the death process through the administered substances. In both cases, an ethical or legal death, whether it is passive euthanasia or physician-assisted suicide requires the consent of the patient or the surrogate person who is either the next-of-kin of the patient or allowed by the courts to make such decision on behalf of the emaciating patient.

HIV/AIDS disclosure Issues in Health Care

Traditionally, HIV/AIDS has been associated with stigmatization, bullying and various stereotypes across the world. This is one of the primary reasons why HIV/AIDS tests are done in private and are often considered highly confidential. Stigmatization of people living with this virus has been rampant and obstructs interventions programs. In addition to this, all patients are entitled to privacy and confidentiality regarding their personal health status at any given time. The difference between other common diseases is that they are widely cured and have been accepted positively by the society, such that it is not an issue when disclosing their details, for instance, a common cold and cancer. AIDS, on the other hand, has traditionally been viewed negatively, until recently. Nonetheless, full disclosure is a personal right (Pozgar, 2013).

Subsequently, the controversy that surrounds AIDS and caregivers is sophisticated. Whereas caregivers are entitled to confidentiality of their HIV status, the patient has the right to know and understand the risks associated with the process. Moreover, doctors have the primary role in curbing the spread of HIV/AIDS. This nurtures a controversy that stretches the right to privacy and confidentiality of the caregiver and the right to quality and risk-free treatment of the patient. Profiling the caregivers according to their HIV/AIDS status amounts to discrimination that eventually lead to stigmatization. Also, placing the patient in the dark regarding the risks involved violates the codes of ethics of the nursing practice (Pozgar, 2013).

Wrongful Conception, Wrongful Birth, and Wrongful Life

Wrongful conception is a medical negligence claim that results in the conception of a healthy child. In other words, the medical carelessness during sterilization procedures of the parents results to the birth or conception of a health unwanted child. Wrongful birth is a claim brought forward by the parents over the medical negligence that causes the birth of an unhealthy child. It occurs when a health practitioner fails to warn the parents about the disabilities of a child before it is born or reaches in advanced stages. Court proceedings allow the compensation of the cost incurred as a result of the child's disabilities. Wrongful life is the term given to a legal action where a severely disabled child sues the parents of health organization for being born, rather than terminating it before he is delivered (Falzon, 2014). The legal litigations can also be initiated against a practitioner or a health center for withholding information regarding the disability, genetic disposition during or before the pregnancy. This concept argues that had the mother or the parents provided with such information at the right time; they would opt for an abortion or other conception methods to avert the birth of a physically challenged child.

Several moral dilemmas result from the above definitions. Pursuing wrongful life and wrongful birth sends a message that physically challenged children are valueless and do have a right to life. In fact, these legal actions suggest that all handicapped children should not be born at all, amounting to profiling, discrimination, and societal immorality. Still, parents have a moral responsibility of guaranteeing their children a comfortable life away from constant suffering, stigmatization and distress as a result of disabilities. Lastly, these actions legalize abortion as a moral concept that can be done at the will of the parents (Falzon, 2014). Such developments might be abused and encourage immorality in the society in case of irresponsible behaviors that lead to unwanted pregnancies.

Partial birth abortions (PBA)

Anti-PBA: Partial birth abortions occur when a baby is delivered up to substantial parts of a living child outside the body of the mother and killing it by sucking the brains followed by crashing of the head. Partial abortion should be banned because it involves deliberate actions of killing the baby, which can survive on its own given better environmental conditions (Koukl, 2013). These procedures are pure murder; why should you bear the pain of giving birth only for someone to kill a living baby? Is it not better if abortion should have been carried out at an earlier stage?

Pro-PBA: The primary term that we should focus on is abortion. Regardless of the stage of fetus development is performed, abortion doesn't make it less impact of the life of the infant. These procedures are sometimes done to protect the life of the mother, especially when the child is disabled and complications have developed. More so, it is the right of women to decide whether or not to carry the pregnancy to full term (Rovner, 2006).

Controversy of Genetic Markers and Stem Cell Research

Notably, one of the major debates regarding stem cell studies comes from the appropriate source of malleable stem cells. Ideally, the human embryo has the highest level of cells that are viable for such activities. Yet, using such sources means the destructions of human embryos. Even though these cells can be harvested during a miscarriage or through donors, encouraging such activities might stimulate inhumanity within the society. This leads to moral and ethical issues of using human embryos as the primary source of stem cells. A majority of religion groups and societies believe that life starts at conception. Therefore, extracting human embryos are equivalent to killing a person deliberately for research purposes (Thomas, 2012).

References

Dworkin,, G. (2008). *Is There a Moral Difference between Passive Euthanasia and Physician-Assisted Suicide? - Euthanasia - ProCon.org. Euthanasia.procon.org.* Retrieved 8 June 2016, from http://euthanasia.procon.org/view.answers.php?questionID=000148

Falzon, C. (2014). *Wrongful Life & Wrongful Birth - Legal and Moral Issues. Academia.edu.* Retrieved 8 June 2016, from https://www.academia.edu/8565869/Wrongful_Life_and_Wrongful_Birth_-_Legal_and_Moral_Issues

Koukl, G. (2013). *Stand to Reason | Partial-Birth Abortion Is Not About Abortion. Str.org.* Retrieved 8 June 2016, from http://www.str.org/articles/partial-birth-abortion-is-not-about-abortion#.V1f4w0B161s

Rovner, J. (2006). *'Partial-Birth Abortion:' Separating Fact from Spin. NPR.org.* Retrieved 8 June 2016, from http://www.npr.org/2006/02/21/5168163/partial-birth-abortion-separating-fact-from-spin

Thomas, I. (2012). *What is the controversy over stem cell research?.* Chicago, Ill: Raintree.

Guido, G. W. (2014). *Legal and ethical issues in nursing*(6th ed.). Upper Saddle River, NJ: Prentice Hall. ISBN: 978-0-1333-5587-1

Pozgar, G. D. (2013). *Legal and ethical issues for health professionals* (3rd ed.). Boston: Jones and Bartlett. ISBN: 978-1-4496-7211-9

YOUR KNOWLEDGE HAS VALUE

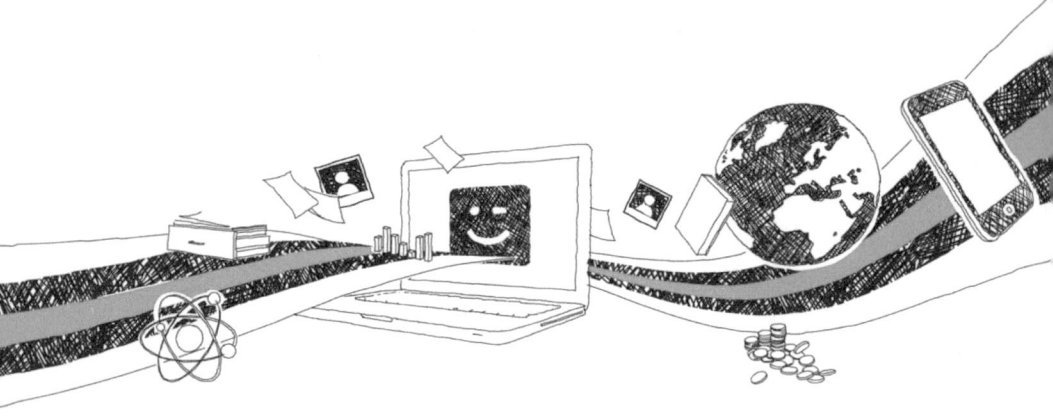

- We will publish your bachelor's and master's thesis, essays and papers

- Your own eBook and book - sold worldwide in all relevant shops

- Earn money with each sale

Upload your text at www.GRIN.com
and publish for free

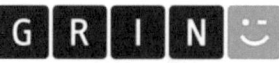